Understanding

PARKII

DISEASE

C000241698

Dr J.M.S. Pearce

Published by Family Doctor Publications
in association with the British Medical Association

IMPORTANT

This book is not intended as a substitute for personal medical advice but as a supplement to that advice for the patient who wishes to understand more about his or her condition.

Before taking any form of treatment YOU SHOULD ALWAYS CONSULT YOUR MEDICAL PRACTITIONER.

In particular (without limit) you should note that advances in medical science occur rapidly and some of the information contained in this booklet about drugs and treatment may very soon be out of date.

© Family Doctor Publications 1995
Reprint 1998, 2000

Family Doctor Publications, 10 Butchers Row, Banbury, Oxon OX16 8JH

Medical Editor: Dr Tony Smith
Consultant Editor: Anne Patterson
Cover Artist: Dave Eastbury
Medical Artist: Angela Christie
Design: Fox Design, Godalming, Surrey
Printing: Reflex Litho, Thetford, Norfolk, using acid-free paper

ISBN: 1 898205 86 8

Contents

AN

ESSAY

ON THE

SHAKING PALSY.

BY

JAMES PARKINSON,

MEMBER OF THE ROYAL COLLEGE OF SURGEONS.

LONDON:

PRINTED BY WHITTINGHAM AND ROWLAND,
Goswell Street,

FOR SHERWOOD, NEELY, AND JONES,

PATERNOSTER ROW.

1817.

James Parkinson (1775–1824), who first described the disease, practised as a GP in Hoxton, a suburb of Shoreditch, London. A great social reformer, author, celebrated biologist and geologist, his 'Essay on the Shaking Palsy', containing descriptions of six of his patients, was published in 1817.

Introduction

If you, or a close relative or friend, suffer from Parkinson's disease, this book is written for you. It is aimed to help you to understand the symptoms and disabilities caused by the disease and to suggest what you can do for yourself as well as what doctors can do to treat the condition. The good news is that, although there is still much to be learned, the grim prospects which prevailed 30 years ago have been improved by increased understanding and modern treatments.

WHAT IS PARKINSON'S DISEASE?

Parkinson's disease is characterised by a collection of signs involving the nervous system, the most important of which are:

- slowness of movement

- rigidity – the limbs may feel heavy and stiff

- shaking (tremor) of the hands and sometimes legs at rest

- disorders of posture – the patient's neck and trunk assume a bent position, and the arms fail to swing freely when walking.

The disease is caused by degeneration of pigmented nerve cells in the brain. It usually starts in the fifties or sixties and can remain stationary for months or years, but usually progresses. Parkinson's disease seldom shortens life expectancy to any significant degree.

In the advanced stages, tremor, slowness and rigidity may affect all four limbs and the trunk; speech may be indistinct and slurred, the limbs and body are bent, and the victim is prone to walk with short, stumbling steps and to fall.

WHO GETS IT?

The illness may afflict people from all classes of society, from all races, and occurs throughout the world. It increases with ageing, but is not caused by ageing itself. Overall, about one person in 1,000 is affected, but this increases to about one in 100 people in their seventies and eighties. Many elderly people are so mildly affected that the condition is easily overlooked. Men and women are equally affected, and the disease is seldom inherited.

Many well-known people, for example, Terry-Thomas and Kenneth More, suffered from the disease and continued a successful, active life for many years.

Don't get too depressed

If this description sounds depressing, remember that for many years, the disability is mild and during this time most patients are capable of normal domestic activities and can usually maintain their normal jobs. Furthermore, although there is no cure for Parkinson's disease, many of the symptoms can be controlled by appropriate treatment.

HOW IS THE DIAGNOSIS MADE?

People wonder how the diagnosis is made. It is invariably a clinical decision, based on the symptoms and especially the signs that the experienced doctor can observe during examination. Laboratory tests and X-rays are generally unnecessary, and special tests such as computed tomography (CT) scans and magnetic resonance imaging (MRI) scans are generally unhelpful; indeed they are often normal in Parkinson's disease.

HOW IS PARKINSON'S DISEASE TREATED?

Treatment is based on the replacement of those chemicals in the brain that are reduced or depleted by Parkinson's disease. The main chemical affected by Parkinson's disease is dopamine, which diminishes slowly for many years before any symptoms are apparent. It is estimated that you have to lose 80 per cent of the dopamine in the critical areas of your brain before symptoms or signs are evident. Dopamine is found in groups of nerve cells in the base of the brain, called the basal ganglia. Patients are given a drug called levodopa to replace the missing dopamine, but other drugs are used too. Levodopa, the drug, is converted to dopamine, the neurotransmitter, in the brain.

Physical therapies

Physical treatment with physiotherapy, and speech and occupational therapy are valuable at certain stages. They supplement, but are not an effective substitute for, drug treatment. The aim throughout is to maintain your activity and as near-normal a lifestyle as possible.

Who will treat you?

Patients and their families have to be as active as the doctors and therapists. Your GP will be the first person to consult and indeed may assume responsibility for managing your condition, including making the diagnosis, explaining and prescribing drugs, and possibly organising physiotherapy and occupational therapy. The GP may then refer you to a consultant, ideally a neurologist, although it could be a general physician or a geriatrician. The consultant will write to your GP confirming the diagnosis and advising him or her about treatment.

Once the diagnosis has been confirmed and treatment started, the GP will provide continuing care, although he or she will probably refer you back to the consultant if any problems arise.

KEY POINTS

✓ Parkinson's disease can affect people from all races and social classes, and men and women are equally affected

✓ The illness is more common in elderly people

✓ Symptoms can be controlled by appropriate treatment

Causes & characteristics

The essential cause is not known. Clues are available from studies of the distribution of the disease, that is, who is affected, where and in what circumstances. These show associations that don't prove a cause, but lead to the investigation of possible causal or contributory factors, which may play a part in causing the illness. I have already mentioned that it is relatively common – perhaps as many as 100,000 patients are affected in the UK at any one time – that men and women are equally affected, and that no race is immune. It is not related to any particular job and is clearly a physical disease of the brain, which is not caused by stress, anxiety, emotional or family upsets. Extensive searches for a viral or bacterial cause have proved negative, so the disease is not infectious.

NERVE CELLS IN THE BRAIN ARE AFFECTED

In patients with Parkinson's disease, there is disease or degeneration of the so-called basal ganglia in the

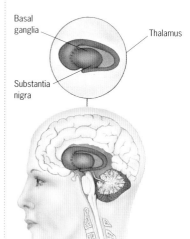

In Parkinson's disease, there is degeneration of the substantia nigra which produces the chemical dopamine deep inside the brain.

deeper grey matter of the brain, particularly of that part known as the substantia nigra.

The substantia nigra, which connects with the striatum (caudate nucleus and globus pallidus), contains black pigmented cells and, in normal individuals, produces a number of chemical transmitters, the most important of which is dopamine. Transmitters are chemicals that transmit, that is, pass on, a message from one cell to the next, either stimulating or inhibiting the function concerned; it is like electricity being the transmitter of sound waves in the radio. Other transmitters include serotonin, somatostatin and noradrenaline. In Parkinson's disease, the basal ganglia cells produce less dopamine, which is needed to transmit vital messages to other parts of the brain, and to the spinal cord, nerves and muscles.

The basal ganglia, through the action of dopamine, are responsible for planning and controlling automatic movements of the body, such as pointing with a finger, pulling on a sock, writing or walking. If the basal ganglia are not working properly, as in Parkinson's disease patients, all aspects of movement are impaired, resulting in the characteristic features of the disease – slowness of movement, stiffness and effort required to move a limb and, often, tremor.

Dopamine levels in the brain's substantia nigra do normally fall with ageing. However, they have to fall to one-fifth of normal values for the symptoms and signs of parkinsonism to emerge.

An important balance

Normally, there is a balance between dopamine and another neurotransmitter – the transmitter of nerve impulses – called acetylcholine. Acetylcholine is present in many areas of the brain and plays a part in normal memory recording and recall. As dopamine is depleted, there is a relative excess of acetylcholine. Thus two of the main groups of drugs used to treat Parkinson's disease are dopamine drugs (levodopa and its preparations Madopar and Sinemet) and drugs designed to restore the balance by diminishing the acetylcholine – anticholinergics (for example, benzhexol [Artane], orphenadrine [Disipal] and benztropine [Cogentin]).

How do the nerve cells send messages?

The diagram on page 6 shows how the nerve cells or neurons in the basal ganglia release packages of the dopamine, transmit it down its main wire or axon, and how this sprouts into receptors of the next nerve cells and transmits the message and nerve impulse further down the line. You can imagine this process carried out by millions of neurons at the same time, forming a network of activity which puts BT and other telephone networks to shame.

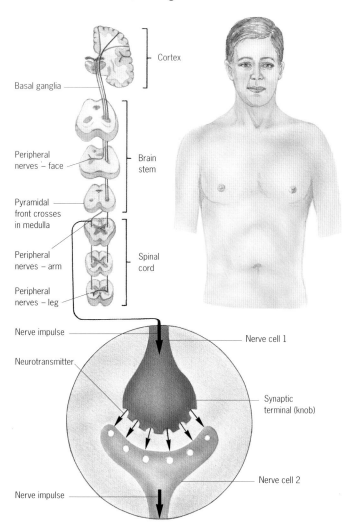

Cortex

Basal ganglia

Peripheral nerves – face

Brain stem

Pyramidal front crosses in medulla

Peripheral nerves – arm

Spinal cord

Peripheral nerves – leg

Nerve impulse

Nerve cell 1

Neurotransmitter

Synaptic terminal (knob)

Nerve cell 2

Nerve impulse

Various parts of the nervous system combine to generate movement. Nerve impulses start in the cortex, pass through the basal ganglia, brain stem and spinal cord, and finally pass through the peripheral nerves which actually control muscles.

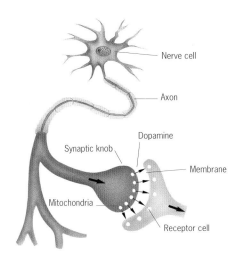

Dopamine is released from storage granules in the nerve cell, and travels down the axon across the synaptic knob to dopamine receptors at the next nerve cell.

Current ideas about the cause of Parkinson's disease suggest a predisposition that makes certain people more vulnerable to some (unidentified) environmental toxic agents. Why cells die in the substantia nigra of Parkinson's disease patients is unknown. This important group of cells shows three changes:

1. Evidence of the release of oxygen compounds by cells which act as a stress that damages cells (oxidative stress), and depletion of a chemical called reduced glutathione.

2. High levels of iron.

3. A deficiency of an essential component of all cells (mitochondrial complex I) that normally controls oxidative reactions; these last involve the release of oxygen compounds which act as stress causing damage to the cells.

Which of these is the primary event, causing secondary changes culminating in death of the nigral cells, is not known. In people with Lewy bodies in their brains but before the development of symptoms of parkinsonism, the substantia nigra shows a comparable loss of reduced glutathione and, possibly, a reduction of complex I activity. Lewy bodies are small areas in nerve cells (inclusions) present in practically every case. They are pink acidophilic (acid-loving) blobs, and show a central core with a peripheral halo. As they may be signs of very early disease, before definite signs emerge, these various abnormalities provide a new focus for the development of future treatments.

Receptors are important

The receptors are most important. Some drugs can block the receptors, and if they are taken for a long period they block the passage of dopamine in the nerve cells and their connecting network of axons. The nerve impulses so essential for normal movements are therefore reduced. This is the basis of the drug-induced parkinsonism I shall describe next.

AGEING AND HEREDITY

Although Parkinson's disease is not caused by the normal ageing process that affects all our brains, just as it does other organs, the incidence of the disease does increase as we get older. The possible role of a genetic abnormality and of hereditary transmission is one of the fertile areas for present and future research. A weak link has been found between Parkinson's disease and Alzheimer's disease, but genetic studies have ruled out any important connection. Nor do the results support any role for genetic factors in the dementia sometimes associated with Parkinson's disease. A family history is obtained in five to ten per cent of patients, but studies on twins suggest that hereditary factors are relatively unimportant. It may be that affected relatives share some environmental agent or are genetically vulnerable to it. What this environmental factor might be, we do not know.

KEY POINTS

✓ The cause of Parkinson's disease is unknown

✓ Research has shown that pigment-containing cells in the deep part of the brain that produce dopamine and other important chemicals degenerate and die. This, in turn, affects the working of other parts of the brain, the spinal cord, nerves and muscles involved in movement

✓ When the chemical dopamine is depleted, there is a relative excess of the chemical acetylcholine

Types of parkinsonism

We separate Parkinson's disease (idiopathic Parkinson's disease or paralysis agitans) described by James Parkinson in 1817 from a group of rarer disorders also caused by impairment of the function of the nerve cells of the brain and called secondary or symptomatic parkinsonism.

There are several kinds of symptomatic parkinsonism:

- drug-induced parkinsonism

- so-called post-encephalitic parkinsonism

- progressive supranuclear palsy

- poison-induced parkinsonism and multi-system atrophies.

It is important to distinguish between true Parkinson's disease and symptomatic parkinsonism because the treatment may be different.

DRUG-INDUCED PARKINSONISM

Neuroleptic drugs used in the treatment of schizophrenia and other serious psychotic mental illnesses can block the release or transmission of dopamine in the substantia nigra and striatum, causing parkinsonism. The most common neuroleptic drugs are the phenothiazines, but there are many others, as shown in the table on page 10. The list is not complete and, if in doubt, you should ask your GP or consultant whether the drug you are taking might cause parkinsonism.

Some of these drugs are used to counter nausea, vomiting or dizziness, and in these circumstances parkinsonism should not develop if the course of treatment is restricted to less than a month for these symptoms. If it is possible for your physician to withdraw the drugs, the parkinsonism will usually slowly disappear, though

DRUGS THAT CAN CAUSE PARKINSONISM

generic name	proprietary name
commonly used neuroleptic drugs:	
chlorpromazine	Largactil
fluphenazine	Moditen, Motival
promazine	Sparine
trifluoperazine	Stelazine
prochlorperazine	Stemetil
thioridazine	Melleril
pericyazine	Neulactil
perphenazine	Fentazin, Triptafen
other similar neuroleptic antipsychotic drugs:	
benperidol	Anquil
droperidol	Droleptan
flupenthixol	Depixol, Fluanxol
zuclopenthixol	Clopixol
haloperidol	Serenace, Haldol, Dozic
reserpine	Serpasil, Decaserpyl
tetrabenazine	Nitoman
sulpiride	Dolmatil
pimozide	Orap
risperidone	Risperdal
those given by injection:	
flupenthixol	Depixol
fluphenazine	Modecate, Moditen
fluspirilene	Redeptin
haloperidol	Haldol
pipothiazine	Piportil

this may take several months. Some patients with serious psychiatric illness need to continue the neuroleptic drugs; some degree of parkinsonism then has to be tolerated to maintain mental stability, and can usually be controlled.

POST-ENCEPHALITIC PARKINSONISM

This type of parkinsonism is now extremely rare. It developed in the wake of a diffuse inflammation of the brain (encephalitis) caused by an epidemic of a particular virus infection which raged throughout the world between 1918 and 1926. The symptoms and treatment are slightly different from those of idiopathic Parkinson's disease.

PROGRESSIVE SUPRANUCLEAR PALSY AND OTHER TYPES OF PARKINSONISM

Parkinsonism is not normally a feature of head injury and is seldom a symptom of a brain tumour. Other disorders, characterised by rigidity and reduced (rigid–akinetic states) can result from a variety of other degenerations of the brain, including the conditions known as progressive supranuclear palsy, multi-system atrophies and Lewy body disease. All these conditions are rare causes of parkinsonism and require specialised neurological assessment; they do not all respond well to anti-parkinsonian drugs:

- Progressive supranuclear palsy is a degenerative condition with limited movements of the eyes, impaired speech and voice, as well as parkinsonism.

- Multi-system atrophies are widespread areas of shrinkage of multiple systems of nerve cells in the brain, in which parkinsonism is preceded or followed by loss of blood pressure, sweating and bladder functions (autonomic dysfunction).

- Lewy body disease is a mixture of parkinsonism with dementia in which there is a high density of Lewy bodies, not only in the deep grey matter but also in the mantle or cortex of the brain.

- Multi-infarct state consists of several areas of softening (infarct) in the brain, the result of multiple strokes. It causes spastic weakness of the limbs and sometimes dementia which may be mistaken for Parkinson's disease.

POISONS-INDUCED PARKINSONISM

It has been found that MPTP, a chemical contaminant of do-it-yourself drugs made illegally and used by heroin addicts, mainly in California, can produce parkinsonism within days or weeks. The brains in fatal cases show severe destruction of the substantia nigra and profound loss of dopamine and other neural transmitters as is seen in Parkinson's disease.

Their symptoms are controlled by levodopa drugs, which replace the missing dopamine in just the same way as in Parkinson's disease. However, the brain damage inflicted by MPTP is permanent. Researchers now have proof that certain poisons can damage the brain in a way similar to that arising spontaneously in idiopathic Parkinson's disease – a valuable finding for further research into the sequence of events leading to degeneration of the dopamine-generating cells.

For example, in animal experiments in which parkinsonism is artificially induced using MPTP, it has been shown that the dopamine-producing cells in the substantia nigra are deficient in one of the important enzymes known as complex I, involved in oxygen control in the cell.

In spite of improved knowledge and understanding of the nature and causes of Parkinson's disease, more work needs to be done to further our knowledge and to develop better treatment.

KEY POINTS

✓ Parkinson's disease needs to be distinguished from various types of symptomatic parkinsonism because the treatment may be different

Symptoms and signs

I have mentioned, earlier, that the principal symptoms of Parkinson's disease are tremor, muscular rigidity, akinesia, abnormal posture and loss of balance. Let's look at these in more detail.

● **Tremor**: the most common early symptom is shaking (tremor) of one or both hands. It occurs at rest and is reduced or stopped when the limb is in action. It is fairly slow – about five beats per second – and is rhythmical. It usually vanishes during sleep.

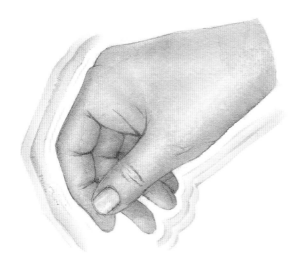

Shaking of one or both hands is the most common early symptom.

- **Rigidity**: by rigidity is meant stiffness and a sense of effort required to move the limb, which may feel heavy and weak. However, loss of strength and power is not a feature of Parkinson's disease.

- **Akinesia**: slowness of movement is experienced in three ways: lack of spontaneous movement (akinesia), slowness in starting a movement, and slowness during the movement (bradykinesia). The handwriting becomes progressively smaller (micrographia: *micro* – small, *graphos* – writing) and may show the tremor.

Dear Dr. Pearce,

This is to authorise you to prepare a report on my medical condition in relation to my ability to drive safely, and to send it to the DVLA.

Characteristically small handwriting of a patient with Parkinson's disease.

- **Disorders of posture**: these refer to the bent position of the neck and trunk that develops late in the disease and describes the way the arms are held close to the sides, elbows and wrists slightly bent; the legs, too, may be flexed at the hips and knees.

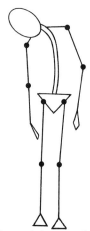

Characteristic posture disorders.

- **Loss of balance**: this commonly accompanies disordered posture. Patients find it difficult to correct a trip or stumble (lack of righting reflexes) and as a consequence are prone to fall. They seem to lean forward in front of their centre of gravity and, without being able to help themselves, a walk may break into a run (called festination by doctors, from the Latin *festinare:* to hurry). Or, if pushed gently, patients may uncontrollably run forwards or stumble backwards.

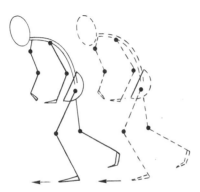

A walk may break into a run. This is called 'festination'.

Symptoms vary a great deal. For example, some patients never develop a tremor.

SIGNS

When your doctor examines you he will notice certain signs, although, as with the symptoms, these vary greatly from patient to patient, and change in the individual at different times. Your movements may be visibly slow (bradykinesia: *brady* – slow, *kinesis* – movement). You may rise slowly from the chair or walk slowly with short steps into the consulting room. You may have a slow rhythmic tremor of one or both arms which disappears on grasping a chair or taking hold of an object. Many years ago this was likened to pharmacists who made pills by rolling them between thumb and index fingers: pill-rolling tremor. When the doctor bends or straightens your wrist or arm or legs he may feel a sense of resistance like trying to bend a lead pipe; he may also feel the tremor superimposed, creating a sensation of turning a cogwheel (known as cogwheel rigidity).

Automatic movements are reduced

Actions are noticeably laboured. Most of us perform automatic movements unconsciously at rest, when sitting comfortably. Such movements, blinking, crossing and uncrossing the legs, and general fidgeting, for example, are lacking in the Parkinson's disease patient. When walking, Parkinson's disease patients use short steps and shuffle, as if the feet are glued to the floor. Gait is hesitant and steps shorten even more in doorways or when there is an obstruction, or if in the street a passing dog or a stranger runs across their path. Sometimes patients get stuck when walking; their feet feel frozen to the ground. If this happens to you, deliberately focus on a spot in front and aim at it with the leading leg: you will find you can usually start to walk again.

Facial appearance and speech are altered

The face may lack expression, the eyes are a little staring, and in advanced cases there is a tendency to dribble saliva. This arises, not because of excessive formation, but because of reduction in the normal swallowing of saliva that we do unconsciously and automatically. The voice is quiet, sometimes hoarse (dysphonia) and the words may be slurred (dysarthria). These problems may be inconspicuous, but may present with difficulty singing in the bath or, more embarrassingly, in the choir.

Bladder and bowel habits change

Constipation is almost invariable. It is caused by sluggish movement of the muscle in the bowel, very similar to that seen in the limbs. It is not a serious symptom, but it does cause much concern and apprehension, particularly in elderly people. Use should be made of over-the-counter medications for controlling constipation. The bladder muscle, too, contracts less efficiently, and frequent calls to pass urine are common, with small volumes and some measure of urgency. In older men, coincidental enlargement of the prostate may add to the problems, with a slow stream and the need to get up at night to pass urine.

If you have these problems, you may need to be assessed by both a neurologist and a urologist. Incontinence does not occur in the early stages of the illness and, if it does occur later, it may have some other explanation. You may have accidents because of physical slowness, being unable to get to the toilet in time; this is not true incontinence but urgency incontinence that can sometimes be improved by drugs such as oxybutynin.

Swallowing may be difficult

Occasionally, difficulty in swallowing develops as a result of the illness, but special tests are

SOME COMMON SYMPTOMS AND SIGNS OF PARKINSON'S DISEASE

- Difficulty fastening buttons
- Can't turn over
- Can't get up from chair
- Expressionless face
- Falls frequently
- Feet freeze
- Greasy skin
- Rarely blinks
- Shuffling steps
- Slow eating
- Slow movement
- Soft voice
- Stiff limbs
- Tremor

needed to make sure this symptom is not due to causes other than parkinsonism, which have arisen by chance.

Some other problems

Usually, these are late features which appear after many years of illness. Most patients are able to walk well, to speak clearly and to work and enjoy leisure activities for many years. Modern specialist treatment by a neurologist controls symptoms effectively in most sufferers.

Other problems occasionally trouble patients. Pain is not a serious problem for most sufferers, though aching and stiffness in the neck, back and limbs is quite common. Because of reduced automatic movement, a stiff or frozen shoulder may develop. This is painful and stops men getting to their wallets in their back trouser pockets and causes women difficulties with zips and bra fasteners. These incidental problems can be treated effectively. Rarely, patients are affected by writer's cramp. Treatment with drugs can also cause symptoms.

KEY POINTS

✓ Symptoms of Parkinson's disease include tremor, rigidity, akinesia, disorders of posture and loss of balance

✓ Symptoms vary a great deal and later in the illness may include changed bladder and bowel habits and difficulty in swallowing

✓ Signs include reduced automatic movements, altered facial appearance and speech

How is the diagnosis made?

Some patients, and even more of their relations, worry about the accuracy of the diagnosis. One patient differs from the next and your symptoms and your appearance may be different from those of the chap shaking away in your local or in the corner shop, who is said to have Parkinson's disease. In most cases an accurate diagnosis is not difficult.

As with certain other diseases, there are no specific or diagnostic tests that confirm or refute the diagnosis. Blood tests, electroencephalograms (EEG), computed tomography (CT) and magnetic resonance imaging (MRI) scans are essentially normal.

Parkinson's disease can be mistaken for other diseases and, because the outlook and treatment may be substantially different, it is generally advisable for the initial suspicion to be confirmed or rejected by a consultant neurologist.

The diagnosis is based on the history and signs and, to the expert eye, may be immediately evident when the patient enters the consulting room. A change in handwriting, dragging of one leg without hip disease or a complaint of clumsiness will all alert the doctor to the possible diagnosis. The severity and the type of illness will be explored in this clinical examination and the disability will be shown by questioning about what you can and cannot do.

WHAT OTHER CONDITIONS LOOK LIKE PARKINSON'S DISEASE?

You can see from the table on page 19 that other causes of shaking and tremors can be mistaken for Parkinson's disease. The most frequent is a common, fairly harmless condition called benign essential tremor, which occurs in two to four per cent of the population, to

CONDITIONS THAT LOOK LIKE PARKINSON'S DISEASE

- Post-encephalitic parkinsonism; drug-induced parkinsonism
- Other causes of tremor – benign essential tremor, thyrotoxicosis, alcoholism
- Other brain disease – multiple strokes

DISEASES NOT TO BE CONFUSED WITH PARKINSON'S DISEASE

- Brain tumour
- Strokes
- Multiple sclerosis
- After-effects of head injury
- Alzheimer's disease and primary dementias
- Motor neuron disease

varying degrees. Here, the shaking is slight or absent at rest but worse when the arms are held stretched out; there is usually no rigidity or slowness of movement and no tendency to a bent or flexed posture. It often, but not always, runs in families, and the tremor may be reduced by a small dose of alcohol. It does not respond to anti-parkinsonian drugs.

Thyroid disease, alcoholism, anxiety states and a variety of rare metabolic and structural disorders can occasionally mimic Parkinson's disease but these will be suspected by the specialist if the symptoms are unusual, and it is only then that investigations may be suggested. These conditions are rarely a diagnostic problem, so tests are not undertaken in most patients.

Multiple sclerosis and strokes

Occasionally, people who are subsequently diagnosed as having Parkinson's disease wonder if it is multiple sclerosis or some form of unusual stroke. Multiple sclerosis is mainly a disease of younger people, and its symptoms and signs are quite different and will be quickly appreciated by the specialist.

Multiple strokes affecting in turn each side of the body can rarely produce a picture that resembles Parkinson's disease superficially; here, expert opinion will separate the two conditions. There is, of course, nothing to prevent both conditions arising by chance in the same unfortunate individual, but the specialist will usually be able to clarify the issue. Strokes do not, however, cause Parkinson's disease.

Is it Alzheimer' s disease?

Sometimes the more advanced or elderly patient may suffer from loss of memory or develop periods of confusion. The family rightly ask: 'Is he becoming demented?' 'Is he developing Alzheimer's disease?' Patients with Alzheimer's disease and the superficially similar Lewy body disease have mental symptoms of forgetfulness and poor judgement from the beginning, whereas in Parkinson's disease the early symptoms are physical slowness, stiffness or tremor. Although the symptoms of Alzheimer's and Parkinson's diseases overlap and resemble each other, neurologists can usually distinguish these conditions on clinical grounds, sometimes supplemented by brain scans and other tests.

KEY POINTS

✓ In most cases an accurate diagnosis is not difficult

✓ Parkinson's disease should not be confused with, and is not caused by, multiple sclerosis or strokes

✓ People with Alzheimer's disease have mental symptoms from the beginning whereas the early symptoms in Parkinson's disease are physical slowness, stiffness or tremor

Does Parkinson's disease affect the mind?

Nervous and emotional factors play their part in all human disease. The effects of worry and sleeplessness in worsening the pain of even a minor bruise or toothache are as well known as the harmful effects of personal worries on the symptoms of, for example, asthma or a stomach ulcer. Conversely, if you have a physical illness such as a broken leg, bronchitis, a breast lump or Parkinson's disease, it is not surprising if you feel anxious, apprehensive or even depressed about it.

The most obvious psychological accompaniments of Parkinson's disease are anxiety or depression caused by the physical symptoms of the disease and the disability it produces. Tremor and ponderous slow movements are a source of social embarrassment. An abnormal gait, trips and falls, difficulty with speech and voice also embarrass the sufferer. At a very late stage, after many years, the physical handicaps can be severe and restrict many activities; it is no wonder that patients then feel despondent and depressed, particularly about their dependence on others. Fears of future incapacity add to their worries.

DEPRESSION

A depressive illness occurs at some time in about one-third of all Parkinson's disease patients. Depressive illness here means symptoms out of proportion to the underlying cause, or symptoms of such severity that the patient can't cope with them. Depression can occur out of the blue when there is no apparent stress, source of anxiety or physical disability to explain it. This is called endogenous depression. It is of interest that the incidence of endogenous depression is higher in people who have developed

Parkinson's disease than in those who do not have the condition. Sometimes it develops before the physical signs of Parkinson's disease are apparent.

Symptoms of depression

If you have ever been depressed you will remember the feelings of being miserable, unhappy and low in spirits; you probably also remember the apathy, being devoid of vitality, interests and enthusiasms. Being depressed is quite different from the common complaint of being bored, anxious or just fed up, so commonly expressed by those who are young, disillusioned and unemployed. Depressed patients have to push themselves to make the effort to do everyday tasks: getting dressed, shaving or putting on make up, going out, mixing socially or even having a chat with family or friends. Life seems pointless, hopeless and futile. Sleep is disturbed. Patients go to bed early, to get away from it all, sleep fitfully till 4 or 5 a.m. and then can sleep no more. Early mornings are the worst time and by evenings the blues may have receded, a little. These diurnal swings of mood are characteristic.

Physical symptoms of vague pains, headaches, backache, palpitations and often a fear of cancer may dominate their lives, adding to the mental miseries. Feelings of wholly inappropriate guilt are mixed with a sense of inadequacy; if you are depressed, you blame yourself for all your family's misfortunes and sometimes for the evils of the world. You will feel periods of restlessness and agitation.

If you feel like this, you need medical attention. Depressed people may commit suicide but this is fortunately rare in Parkinson's disease.

Treating depression is worthwhile

Symptoms generally respond well to antidepressant drugs of the tricyclic group (amitriptyline, dothiepin, etc.) but they must be supervised by your GP or specialist. They do not interact with anti-parkinsonian drugs. Newer antidepressive drugs are of equal value and include the much-publicised paroxitene (Prozac). Treatment is usually necessary for six to twelve months, sometimes longer. Results are generally good.

CONFUSION AND HALLUCINATIONS

These symptoms are uncommon both in younger patients and in the early stages of the disease. Don't forget that many people over the age of 70 have periods of memory lapses, disorientation and confusion. Deafness and impaired vision can lead to hallucinations in people without Parkinson's disease.

When they occur in Parkinson's disease they may be the result of ageing effects alone, or they may be caused by drugs, or by the parkinsonian effects on the brain. Antiparkinsonian drugs of all types may cause disorientation, confusion and hallucinations. The most common ones are anticholinergic drugs, for example, benzhexol (Artane), orphenadrine (Disipal), benztropine (Cogentin), but bromocriptine (Parlodel) and levodopa drugs (Madopar, Sinemet) can also cause confusional states. Confusion, disorientation or hallucinations may result.

What happens?

Nightmares and frequent dreams are early warnings of these unpleasant side effects. In most instances these problems come and go intermittently, but always tend to be more noticeable at night, in strange surroundings, such as hospitals or nursing homes. Disorientation may be related to time, place or person. The patient is bewildered and does not know where she or he is, or what time of day it is. Recent information is imperfectly registered, so that the patient may deny having had lunch an hour ago, or forget having seen a recent visitor.

Visual hallucinations consist of seeing things that are not there: seeing people, faces, insects or animals. Auditory hallucinations consist of hearing sounds or voices that are not there: a radio or TV may seem to emit voices or they may seem to come from inside the patient's head. Sometimes the victim knows they are unreal, but having insight into these intrusions sometimes he or she may believe them to be real. They can cause distress and agitation.

Confusion may betray itself in peculiar conversations or strange erratic behaviour. Patients may wander off and get lost. They are often inattentive, distractible and memory appears poor because they seem unable to concentrate. Alternatively, they might pour milk into the teapot, put on clothes back to front, attempt to eat puddings with a knife or find themselves unable to tie a knot in their tie, or to use a comb or razor. These latter difficulties are technically called apraxia: the inability to perform skilled movements and sequences when the limbs have normal powers of strength, coordination and sensation.

Drug effects

Although these symptoms may occur in demented patients and are often not totally curable, they may just be a sign of sensitivity to drugs. The doctor will reduce or gradually tail off any possible offending drug and symptoms will generally disappear. Obviously, reduction of anti-parkinsonian treatment may lead to an increase in the slowness and rigidity of the disease, but in the end it is easier to handle a sane but physically slow patient than a more mobile confused one. A fine balance of drugs, tailored to the individual's needs, will often provide a satisfactory if not perfect solution.

DEMENTIA

One of the big worries about Parkinson's disease is that it is known to be associated with dementia – a decline in intellect, memory and the ability to make rational decisions and judgements. This has, without doubt, been overemphasised. Many parkinsonian patients are not affected in this way and never become demented.

In later life both Parkinson's disease and Alzheimer's disease, the most frequent cause of dementia, are common. At the age of 70, about five to ten per cent of the population show some signs of dementia, and about half of these will suffer from Alzheimer's disease. Thus there is a chance that some patients, purely by coincidence, have both parkinsonism and dementia.

The combination is obviously unfortunate and the outlook is considerably worse. Coincidence apart, it is known that about 10 to 20 per cent of Parkinson's disease patients will develop dementia. If the dementing illness is apparent at the outset, the outlook is worse. If such patients are given levodopa drugs for their parkinsonian symptoms, they can tolerate only small doses, and are prone to side effects, particularly confusional states and hallucinations. In other words, dementia limits the amount of levodopa it is possible to give, and the control of parkinsonian symptoms is less satisfactory for this reason.

The combination of Parkinson's disease and dementia is ultimately disabling. Families will need all the welfare services possible to cope with the patient at home. Ultimately, periods in longer-term hospitals or private nursing homes may be necessary. Research in this very difficult area is active and there is every hope that progress will be made.

KEY POINTS

✓ People with Parkinson's disease often feel anxious, apprehensive or even depressed about their illness

✓ Medical attention is needed early in depression

✓ Confusions and hallucinations may be caused by sensitivity to anti-parkinsonian drugs, or by other unrelated illnesses

✓ The combination of Parkinson's disease and dementia makes treatment difficult

Disability in Parkinson's disease

If you have just been told that you have Parkinson's disease, I expect you will feel gloomy and despondent. You will have visions of a shuffling, bent old person, see yourself in a wheelchair and feel disheartened by the possibility of your family and friends having to look after your every need. These feelings are common, but in many cases they are unjustified by subsequent events.

GETTING THINGS IN PERSPECTIVE

It is important to understand the illness and to get it into perspective. Whereas it is true that some patients do end up with severe physical and mental disabilities, many do not. A lot depends on how old you are when the condition is first noticed. If, for instance, you have been fit and reasonably active and when you are, say, 74 you

develop a shaking in one hand and a little stiffness and slowness of movement in that arm, we can safely say that your life expectation won't be reduced, and that the parkinsonian symptoms are unlikely to cause much disability before you are in your eighties; even then, they may not be serious. Other coincidental illnesses – arthritis, bronchitis, heart disease and strokes – are more likely to cause difficulties.

If you are one of those afflicted when unusually young, say in your thirties or forties, the rate of worsening is often slow and, although severe physical problems are eventually likely, you will probably have many years of good function and be able to continue with your work and home life. Moreover, new modifications of treatment develop so quickly that the outlook may well be much better during the next decade.

DETERIORATION IS OFTEN SLOW

In general the course of the illness is a slow one. Sudden deterioration is unlikely unless brought about by other illness or by use of the wrong drugs. In my experience and that of others, the disease remains stationary for five, ten or more years, in as many as perhaps 15 to 20 per cent of patients, and disabilities are mild and do not increase during this period. Why this is so, we do not know.

IS THE TREATMENT WORKING?

The effects of treatment are vitally important in determining how much trouble the illness causes. The effects of treatment are usually most gratifying for several years. In order to assess how effective treatment is, or the stage of the disease at any one time, it is helpful to record the main problems, signs and disabilities. This is done in the consulting room. However, we also have several scales for classifying the stages of the illness. Overall severity is rated on the established, but probably over-simplified, Hoehn and Yahr scale (named after the individuals who developed it).

There are also detailed scales describing problems in walking, feeding, dressing and other activities of daily living (ADL). The lengthy Unified Parkinson's Disease Rating Scale (UPDRS), the King's College Hospital Scale and the North Western University Disability Scale are also in common use.

The Webster Score is a simpler scale for assessment, and takes only five to ten minutes. It is used by doctors to record slowness of movement (bradykinesia), rigidity, tremor, gait, speech and so on. It comprises 10 items graded 0 to 3 each, producing scores of 0 (no signs of disability) to a maximum of 30 (most severe). There are two

HOEHN AND YAHR SCALE FOR RATING SEVERITY OF DISABILITY

Five stages have been arbitrarily assigned:

Stage I   Unilateral disease only
Stage II Bilateral mild disease
Stage III Bilateral disease with early impairment of postural stability
Stage IV Severe disease requiring considerable assistance
Stage V   Confinement to bed or wheelchair unless aided

WEBSTER SCORE FOR PARKINSON'S DISEASE

Each item is graded according to a specific schedule which is scored 0 to 3. See Glossary (page 59) for explanation of terms.

1. Bradykinesia of hands
2. Rigidity
3. Posture
4. Arm swing
5. Gait
6. Tremor
7. Facies
8. Seborrhoea
9. Speech
10. Self-care

TOTAL: /30
Date:
Time:

Additional items suggested (scored 0–3, 1 point each):

Balance
Rising from chair
Dyskinesia

MENTAL STATE (scored 0–3)

Confusion
Hallucinosis
Dementia

---

additional useful features: a check on balance and the ability to get up from a chair. There are also scales for assessing dyskinesia (jerky, twitching movements).

The chart on page 29 may be helpful in assessing your progress periodically and the effects of treatment.

You will see that by repeated use of these scales it is possible to measure the degree of improvement resulting from any form of treatment.

Just as the quality of life has been enhanced by drug treatment, so has the duration of life. Before the levodopa drugs, the life expectancy was about 12 years. Many parkinsonian patients now have a normal life expectancy and are more likely to succumb to unrelated, common illnesses that affect elderly people.

DYSKINESIA SCALES

A. Duration: the time when dyskinesia is present during waking hours:

0 = none
1 = 1 to 25 per cent of waking hours
2 = 26 to 50 per cent
3 = 51 to 75 per cent
4 = 76 to 100 per cent

B. Severity of dyskinesia

0 = noticeable, mild but not disabling
1 = mildly disabling
2 = moderately disabling
3 = severely disabling

Note: additional scales can be made 0 to 3 for painful dyskinesia, and for dystonias

DAILY PARKINSONISM MONITORING CHART

Check with the key below, then please fill in hourly

Name:

	7am	8am	9am	10am	11am	12pm	1pm	2pm	3pm	4pm	5pm	6pm	7pm	8pm	9pm	10pm
Mobility	2/e/md	1	1	1	1	2	3/md	2	1	1	2	2	2/md	2	1	1
Tremor	+	–	–	–	–	+	++	–	–	–	–	++	+	–	–	–
Dyskinesia	–	++	–	–	–	+	–	++	–	–	–	–	–	+	–	–

Mobility key
1. Walks unaided
2. Walks with help of one
3. Cannot walk

T. Resting parkinsonian tremor +/++/+++
D. Dyskinesia +/++/+++

Drug key
ap = apomorphine
art = benzhexol (Artane)
br = bromocriptine (Parlodel)
dis = orphenadrine (Disipal)
e = selegiline (Eldepryl)
ly = lysuride
md = Madopar
sin = Sinemet

KEY POINTS

✓ Not all Parkinson's disease patients end up with severe physical and mental disabilities

✓ Specially designed scales are used to assess the severity of disability and the impact of treatment

✓ Many patients now have a normal life expectancy

Medical treatment

Treatment is aimed at abolishing as far as possible the symptoms and disabilities caused by the illness. We do not yet have any drugs that will cure the disease or affect the natural progression. What the available drugs will do is to reverse the symptoms by replacing the essential chemicals, such as dopamine, necessary for normal transmission of nerve impulses and control of movements.

KEY FEATURES OF TREATMENT

- Treatment should be tailor-made to suit the needs of each individual, and will need adjustments of fine-tuning at intervals over the entire course of the illness. In Parkinson's disease it is not enough to put the patient on one tablet, three times per day, and leave it at that!

- Treatment should always be governed by symptoms and by disability. For example, at the onset, when symptoms may be mild and inconspicuous, it is often best to give no drugs at all.

- Correct management means more than drugs alone. Active and positive efforts are necessary from you and from any available relatives. Help is also needed from general practitioners, physiotherapists, occupational therapists and various welfare services at certain times in the disease.

Who will treat you?

In my view, most patients should be referred to a hospital specialist – usually a neurologist – at an early stage in order to confirm the diagnosis and to obtain advice about the immediate and future prospects of treatment. Patients are seen at intervals to assess their progress and drug treatment. Thereafter, the neurologist will arrange for regular follow-up at intervals which vary from two months to a year.

Increasingly, GPs are continuing treatment for patients, but obviously should refer them to the consultant if problems develop.

DRUG TREATMENT

I have already described the deficiency of essential dopamine in the brain and the excess of acetylcholine relative to the dopamine, that occurs in Parkinson's disease. Thus, early treatment consists of drugs called anticholinergics, which diminish acetylcholine and restore the balance with dopamine.

Later, amantadine may be introduced; this substance has mild dopamine-releasing properties, boosting dopamine levels; it is weakly anticholinergic and has few side effects.

Agonists are agents that drive or stimulate the working of the site or receptor on which they act. Some neurologists introduce dopamine agonists (pergolide or bromocriptine) next, because they cause less jerky, twitching movements (dyskinesia) than does the drug most often used for established disease, namely levodopa. However, within the first three to four years, most patients do need a levodopa drug.

Levodopa is converted to active dopamine. The old pure levodopa has now been replaced by combinations of levodopa with carbidopa (Sinemet) or levodopa with benserazide (Madopar). Carbidopa and benserazide concentrate the dopamine in the brain and allow a reduction of dosage and side effects. These drugs are the mainstay of drug treatment and more effective than other drugs currently available. Several drugs are available as syrups and elixirs for patients who have difficulty swallowing tablets or capsules. The striking benefits afforded by these drugs may, in some cases, slowly wear off after five to ten years, but still offer some relief of symptoms. Patients' needs and responses to therapy vary widely, so do not take too literally the dosages or regimens mentioned here.

If the levodopa drugs are not adequate, another group of drugs, called dopamine agonists, may be used. They stimulate the dopamine receptors rather than supply more dopamine; pergolide, bromocriptine and lysuride are examples.

Sometimes, apomorphine, described on page 38, is used, but this has to be administered by regular injections, rather like a diabetic patient using insulin. It has the great advantage of giving about one hour's (50 to 90 minutes) benefit starting within five to ten minutes of the injection; this is useful in helping you to handle a pressing social or business engagement.

Selegiline is itself a weak anti-parkinsonian drug but is valuable in early disease to control symptoms and delay by about one year the use of Madopar or Sinemet. Its use is described in a later section. Selegiline also reduces the wearing off of the effects of Madopar and Sinemet which occurs in the later stages of the disease (end-of-dose akinesia).

Anticholinergic drugs

These are valuable for treating early tremor and rigidity but are not as potent as levodopa in treating slowness, freezing and falls. They are good at controlling salivation and drooling, because they cause a dry mouth. They work well with levodopa drugs, but are generally tailed off gradually in older patients or if there is any tendency to confusion, hallucinations or memory impairment. Symptoms from an enlarged prostate gland or any liability to glaucoma may be worsened.

Anticholinergic drugs are particularly helpful in drug-induced parkinsonian states and in the now rare post-encephalitic cases. There is little to choose between the various drugs shown in the table in terms of potency or side effects.

Levodopa drugs

These are the treatment of choice for moderate and severe Parkinson's disease. Rigidity, slowness, posture and often tremor are improved by levodopa drugs. In elderly people, they are less useful because a dose sufficient to benefit the symptoms tends to cause unacceptable side effects. Carefully supervised use of low doses is advisable on a trial or error basis. They should not generally be used in parkinsonism induced by neuroleptic drugs, and produce only unpredictable and limited benefit in parkinsonism secondary to degenerative diseases (see pages 9–11).

ANTICHOLINERGIC DRUGS

Drug	Trade name	Single dose per tablet or capsule	Dose range per day
Orphenadrine	Disipal	50 mg	100–300 mg
	Biorphen (syrup/elixir)	25 mg/5 ml	
Benzhexol	Artane	2 or 5 mg	6–15 mg
	Broflex (syrup)	5 mg/5 ml	
Benztropine	Cogentin	2 mg	1–4 mg
Procyclidine	Kemadrin	5 mg	7.5–30 mg
	Arpicolin (syrup)	2.5 mg/5 ml and 5 mg/5 ml	

LEVODOPA-DERIVED DRUGS

Drug	Trade name	Single dose (per tablet or capsule)	Dose of levodopa tablet per day
Levodopa with benserazide	Madopar	62.5/125/250 mg	100–800 mg
	Madopar CR	125 mg	100–1200 mg
Levodopa with carbidopa	Sinemet	110/275 mg	100–800 mg
	Sinemet LS	62.5 mg	
	Sinemet plus	125 mg	
	Half Sinemet CR	125 mg	100–1,200 mg
	Sinemet CR		100–1,200 mg

Drug dose is gradually increased

Treatment is started with a small dose, taken with food, two or three times per day. This is gradually increased until the smallest dose necessary to produce acceptable control of symptoms and disability is reached; it usually takes six to twelve weeks to produce a stable state of control.

Drugs such as Sinemet and Madopar contain a mixture of levodopa and a second drug that concentrates the levodopa in the brain and minimises side effects elsewhere in the body.

For example, Sinemet 110 contains 100 milligrams (mg) levodopa plus 10 mg carbidopa; Madopar 250 contains 200 mg levodopa plus 50 mg benserazide.

Balancing benefit against side effects

The best dose is often a compromise between almost-total control of all symptoms and side effects. Many physicians like to keep a little in reserve for future needs. Most patients are untroubled by early side effects, although occasionally nausea, vomiting and fainting are a nuisance; these are easily overcome by dose adjustments and timing.

Unwanted side effects

After one or two years, some patients develop abnormal jerky, twitching (choreic) or writhing (athetoid) movements called drug-induced dyskinesia. They occur one to three hours after a dose when brain levels of dopamine are at their peak. They affect the mouth, tongue, lips and cheeks, and often the neck, limbs and trunk. They more often trouble the patient's partner than the patients themselves, for they are embarrassing and unsightly rather than disabling. If severe, they can be reduced or abolished by smaller doses of the drugs, which may then need to be given more frequently. The patient with dyskinesia on Sinemet 275, three times a day, may be relieved of it by Sinemet 110 in five or six doses at intervals of two to three hours. The usual response of Parkinson's disease and other kinds of symptomatic parkinsonism to levodopa and anticholinergic drugs is shown in the table on page 37.

Wearing-off effects

At a later stage of Parkinson's disease the duration of action of drugs seems shorter. You may notice wearing off at the end of each dose (end-of-dose akinesia) before the next tablets are due, or you may be aware of wearing off on waking each morning (early morning akinesia) because the last evening's dose has worn off. Slowness, stiffness and freezing are the most troublesome features. Sometimes a dose seems to fail to work, often an after-lunch dose. This is sometimes caused by proteins in the stomach and intestine, from the preceding meal, interfering with the absorption of the drug into the bloodstream. Modifying the diet may improve this problem (see page 54).

The recently developed slow-release (controlled-release or CR) preparations are useful in some patients. A single dose in the evening may reduce the troublesome difficulties of turning over in bed, or getting up to the lavatory. It may

DRUG TREATMENT OF PARKINSON'S DISEASE ACCORDING TO STAGE OF DISEASE

Symptoms and disability	Treatment
No disability	No drugs or selegiline
Symptoms a nuisance/ embarrassment	Anticholinergics* and/or selegiline
Stiff and slow despite anticholinergics	Add amantadine or pergolide
Slow, marked tremor, falls, work in jeopardy	Levodopa given as Madopar or Sinemet
Early dyskinesia or fluctuations	Smaller doses often + pergolide
Late levodopa failure	Long-acting Madopar or Sinemet + pergolide, or apomorphine injections

*Not in elderly or confused people.
Pergolide, bromocriptine and lysuride are alternative, similar drugs.
Note: combinations of drugs are often used

SIDE EFFECTS OF LEVODOPA-DERIVED DRUGS

Early (in first few days and weeks)	Nausea, vomiting, fainting: all wear off within a few weeks
Late (after 1–3 years)	Wearing-off at end of dose Dyskinesia and dystonia 'On–off' fluctuations Mental confusion, hallucinations

also control dystonic cramps in the legs and feet, and may give greater mobility on waking, before the first dose of ordinary levodopa is given.

The single dose of a CR preparation at night needs to be used with the usual daytime regimen of ordinary Madopar or Sinemet. An alternative regimen is to take the CR preparation alone, regularly in the daytime, in place of the usual levodopa drugs; the levels of drug in the blood and brain tend to be lower and achieved more slowly. The dose needs to be increased by about 50 per cent above the previous levodopa dosage. This produces a more smooth and even response of symptoms and shorter periods of immobility in the 'off' phase. However, many patients find that they are never fully active or 'on', and prefer the usual shorter-acting Sinemet or Madopar.

'On–off' episodes

Later, 'on–off episodes' may develop. The 'on' phase occurs at peak dose and the patient is then mobile and independent, but often has abnormal dyskinetic movements. The 'off' phase consists of sudden freezing, feet sticking to the floor and immobility, sometimes with a feeling of fear and panic. Patients may suddenly switch from 'on' to 'off' and from 'off' to 'on' 'like switching on a light switch'. This is disconcerting and may be wrongly thought to be nervous or psychologically caused. Smaller, more frequent doses may ease this difficult problem.

A related problem is painful cramp-like twisting of the ankle and toes that occurs often at the end of the dose – just before the next dose is due, or sometimes at night. This is called drug-induced dystonia.

You will appreciate that all these drug manipulations require patience and skill from both patient and physician. It is often necessary to admit such patients to hospital for specialised care, frequent checks and ratings of symptoms, side effects and dosage in order to achieve the fine-tuning for optimal

RESPONSE OF PARKINSON'S DISEASE AND OTHER KINDS OF SYMPTOMATIC PARKINSONISM TO LEVODOPA AND ANTICHOLINERGIC DRUGS

Condition	Levodopa	Anticholinergic drugs
Parkinson's disease	+++	++
Drug-induced parkinsonism	++	++
Multi-system atrophies, including progressive supranuclear palsy	+/–	+/–
Other causes of parkinsonism	+/–	+/–

+++ usually very good
++ moderate
+ some
+/– variable response

performance. This may take one to two weeks.

Other side effects

The other important unwanted effects are mental disturbances, such as confusion, disorientation, and failing memory and concentration. As you grow older, abnormal movements or mental disturbances may make it necessary to reduce the dosage of levodopa. This may make you much calmer and more contented, but it is likely to increase your parkinsonian features – slowness and rigidity, the difficulties in walking, posture and falls. In the end, most families find it easier to handle a patient who is slow, perhaps immobile, but rational than one who is more active, but disorientated and confused.

DOPAMINE AGONISTS

It is fashionable to introduce these drugs at an early stage, before levodopa, because they cause less dyskinesia than levodopa, and it is thought that they may delay the appearance of levodopa dyskinesias and fluctuations. Another use is to introduce a dopamine agonist when dyskinesia, mental side effects or 'on–off' fluctuations develop. It is then helpful to add a dopamine agonist, which stimulates or excites the dopamine receptors into greater activity. This addition allows a small reduction in levodopa dose, thus diminishing the side effects.

Pergolide, bromocriptine and lysuride are similar dopamine agonist drugs. Patients with severe vascular, kidney or liver disease, or those who are pregnant or breast-feeding, should not generally take this group of drugs because of possible adverse side effects.

These dopamine agonists are started in small doses and slowly increased every week or so until benefit is apparent without undue side effects. It may take two or three months until the best stable dose is found. If they are added to Sinemet or Madopar, when the benefit begins it may be possible to reduce the levodopa dose by about 25 per cent.

Side effects

Dopamine agonists are strong drugs, which reduce all the symptoms of Parkinson's disease, but their side effects can be prohibitive. They cause more severe psychiatric complications of confusion, delusions and frank aggressive behaviour in a number of patients. These are usually reversible on reducing the dose, but often it is necessary to stop the drug. These psychiatric complications are especially likely in the over-70s and in those with previous confusion or dementia. Dopamine agonists can also aggravate stomach ulcers and arterial disease in the legs. In general they should not be given to older patients, and should always be supervised by a specialist.

Apomorphine

This is an old drug that has found a new use. It, too, is a dopamine agonist, but it has to be given by a pump or by injections subcutaneously (under the skin) in the lower abdomen or outer thigh, which many patients or relatives can be taught to give. It causes vomiting unless each dose is preceded by domperidone, a potent anti-vomiting drug taken by mouth.

Apomorphine injections can be

DOPAMINE AGONISTS

Drug	Trade name	Single dose	Dose/day
Bromocriptine	Parlodel	1, 2.5, 5, 10 mg	20–100 mg
Lysuride	Revanil	200 micrograms (µg)	600–5,000 µg
Pergolide	Celance	50, 250, 1,000 µg*	750–4,000 µg
Apomorphine	Britaject	10 mg in 2 ml ampoule	3–30 mg
Cabergoline	Cabaser	1, 2, 4 mg	2–6 mg
Ropinirole	Requip	0.25, 1, 2, 5 mg	3–9 mg

*Note: 1,000 micrograms (µg) = 1 milligram (mg).

helpful, giving about one hour's (50 to 90 minutes) almost certain benefit starting within five to ten minutes of the injection. This is useful if you have an important social or business engagement. The injections can be repeated two or three times each day, under specialist advice. Dyskinesia can result if the dose is too high, and the correct dose for you has to be found by trial and error, always starting with a small dose.

NEWER DRUGS

The search for more effective medications for Parkinson's disease is likely to be aided by the recent isolation of at least five individual brain receptors for dopamine. There are newer dopamine agonists – ropinirole, pramipexole and cabergoline. These drugs mimic the role of dopamine in the brain, stimulating the dopamine receptor neurons. They are slightly less effective than levodopa in controlling rigidity and bradykinesia. Their main use is in patients in whom levodopa is no longer effective, or who cannot tolerate adequate dosage. Used with small doses of levodopa, they may reduce fluctuations in performance and shorten the 'off' periods in the later stages. Their use is also often limited by side effects, including hallucinations, confusion, dyskinesias, nightmares, nausea and vomiting, and vascular complications.

Ropinirole (Requip) is a dopamine agonist that controls symptoms of Parkinson's disease. Its side effects are similar to those of the older dopamine agonists. They can all be used as single therapy (monotherapy) in some younger patients for control of symptoms, which permits a delay of a year or two before introducing levodopa. Thus, it delays for a time the dyskinesias of treatment with dopamine. In more advanced disease, they are usually given with levodopa to bolster the effect of smaller doses of levodopa. The dose is initially 0.25 milligrams (mg), one tablet three times a day, increased by 0.75 mg at weekly intervals to a maximum dose of 3–9 mg/day, that is, 3,000 to 9,000 μg/day.

Pramipexole (Mirapexin): in clinical trials, patients taking pramipexole alone saw as much as a 30 per cent improvement in symptoms. Combining pramipexole with levodopa drugs allowed disabled patients to reduce levodopa doses by up to 25 per cent. The initial dose is one 88-mg tablet three times a day, then doubling the dose every week to a maximum of 3.3 mg/day. Some patients develop a fall in blood pressure with fainting during the first few days of therapy, and should be warned of this if driving or operating machinery. It is a non-ergot dopamine agonist with moderate anti-parkinsonian activity.

OTHER DRUGS

Drug	Trade name	Dose	Dose/day
Amantadine	Symmetrel	100 mg	200 mg
Selegiline	Eldepryl	10 mg	5–10 mg
	Eldepryl Syrup	10 mg/5 ml	

Apart from avoiding the ergot-type vascular effects, its side effects are similar to those of other dopamine agonists. It is used as an alternative dopamine agonist.

Cabergoline (Cabaser) has the advantage of a long duration of action – more than 24 hours. In comparison, pramipexole lasts for about eight hours. The dose is one 1-mg tablet daily, increased by weekly increments of 0.5–1.0 mg/day to 2–6 mg. Some patients develop a fall in blood pressure with fainting during the first few days of therapy, and should be warned of this if driving or operating machinery.

COMT inhibitors (entacapone)

Although well short of a cure, catechol methyltransferase (COMT) inhibitors represent an entirely new class of therapy that will help many Parkinson's disease patients obtain better symptom control. As they have no effect on symptoms of Parkinson's disease when given alone, the COMT inhibitors are used in combination with levodopa to increase its duration of action. They do so by blocking catechol-O-methyltransferase, an enzyme that metabolises levodopa. Thus, more levodopa is available for conversion to dopamine in the brain. The first of these drugs, tolcapone, has been withdrawn because of unwanted side effects. Clinical trials suggest that entacapone is also especially helpful for reducing motor fluctuations in patients with advanced Parkinson's disease. It appears to be well tolerated.

SELEGILINE (ELDEPRYL)

This is a weak anti-parkinsonian drug, but it slightly strengthens the effects of levodopa drugs and it may reduce the 'on–off' swings, especially the immobility in the 'off' phase. It is best given early in the illness, and is useful because it controls most of the early symptoms for one to two years.

The early reports that selegiline had a protective effect, slowing down the disease, have sadly proved to be untrue. A single dose of 10 mg each morning is well tolerated, and side effects are not common.

One group of UK researchers has found a small increased mortality rate and a tendency to fainting attacks (syncope) in some patients treated with selegiline, although most published series do not show any such effects. No reason for this has been shown and, as a causal link is not yet established, most physicians continue to use the drug in standard dosage.

DRUG HOLIDAYS

In resistant cases with random 'on–off' swings and poor control of parkinsonian symptoms, drug holidays have been tried. The aim is that, by withdrawal of drugs, an attempt is made to rest or to reset the dopamine receptors that have been overdriven by levodopa and other drugs, and to rid the brain of theoretical toxic byproducts of these drugs. This is all unproven speculation and, in practice, benefits only sufferers who are plainly overdosed.

Restabilisation is then necessary, in hospital with hourly recording charts of parkinsonian signs, disability, mental performance and side effects. These observations usually reveal the problem, and then we often stop inessential or weak-acting drugs and those medications thought to be unnecessary for coincidental ailments. The dose of levodopa is reduced by 50 to 75 per cent and, as side effects disappear, drugs are reintroduced gradually until the smallest effective dose is found. Simplification is the hallmark of effective treatment.

In difficult cases, it is sometimes helpful to apply an apomorphine or levodopa test dose. A single high dose is given after a 24-hour period of drug withdrawal, and the effects give a good indication of whether or not the dopamine receptors are still responsive. If they are not, there is plainly no sense in persisting with dopaminergic (dopamine-acting) drugs. The test gives important information that predicts future responses to treatment. A single dose of 250 mg Madopar or an injection of two to ten mg apomorphine will demonstrate dopamine responsiveness by showing improvement of at least 20 per cent in one of the standard rating scales I discussed earlier.

SOME DRUG WARNINGS

Certain drugs should not be used in Parkinson's disease. I have mentioned the major phenothiazine tranquillisers and anti-psychotic drugs (neuroleptics). These drugs may also be suggested for nausea or for dizzy attacks but should seldom be used in Parkinson's disease. Monoamine oxidase inhibitors used for depression are not allowed, but tricyclic antidepressants are in order. Patients with certain types of glaucoma or skin melanoma should not take levodopa drugs because they may worsen these conditions.

Vitamin B$_6$ (pyridoxine), present in multi-vitamin capsules and medicines, and used for premenstrual tension, blocks the action of levodopa, but there is no interaction if given with Sinemet or Madopar. If in doubt, you should always consult your doctor.

NEW TREATMENT APPROACHES

In addition to new drugs there are other new approaches to treatment.

Gene therapy holds considerable potential for the treatment of central nervous system disease. The introduction of functional genes into the brain of patients with Parkinson's disease may prove useful as a means to replace a defective gene. It aims to introduce a protein, which can protect against cell damage or restore the workings of a damaged cell, or permit the physiological delivery of a deficient neurotransmitter. The strategies for gene therapy techniques have expanded beyond the classic dopamine replacement towards the use of factors that induce nerve cell growth (neurotrophic factors) in enhancing cell function or preventing cell death.

KEY POINTS

✓ Drug treatment reverses the symptoms of Parkinson's disease by replacing the essential chemicals necessary for normal transmission of nerve impulses and control of movements

✓ Drugs are chosen to match the stage of the disease and need adjustments at intervals over the entire course of the illness

✓ Pure levodopa has been replaced by combinations of levodopa with carbidopa (Sinemet) or levodopa with benserazide (Madopar). These are the most effective drugs currently available

✓ Unwanted side effects can be reduced or abolished by altering the drug dose

✓ When wearing-off effects of drugs are troublesome, the recently developed slow-release (controlled release or CR) preparations are useful in a few patients

✓ Dopamine agonists should not be given to older patients and should always be supervised by a specialist

Surgery for Parkinson's disease

This consists of destruction of tiny parts of the brain (stereotactic surgery and pallidotomy), electrical stimulation of small parts of the brain (deep brain stimulation) or transplantation of dopamine-producing tissue into the brain.

STEREOTACTIC SURGERY

Thirty years ago there was a vogue for placing tiny destructive lesions in the basal ganglia by means of a stereotactic apparatus, which permitted very accurate placement of the lesion. This was fairly effective in controlling tremor and rigidity – if it was one-sided. Stereotactic surgery is of no benefit in correcting facial expression, weak voice, slowness of movement, stooped posture and tendency to fall. Indeed, sometimes these symptoms are made worse.

Stereotactic surgery is still used, especially for early one-sided tremor and rigidity, if they fail to respond to other measures. In most specialised centres in the UK and the USA, however, it is seldom used because levodopa drugs, despite their shortcomings, have in general proved so effective. Occasional patients may benefit from such operations if their main problem is one-sided shaking and rigidity that cannot be controlled by drug treatment. The decision requires expert neurological advice. New techniques are being developed, but require time before their benefits and risks can be fully assessed. Stereotactic gamma thalamotomy has met with some success, reducing rigidity and also tremor in otherwise resistant cases. It consists of using gamma radiation aimed at destroying a tiny part of the thalamus, which is a central part of the basal ganglia.

PALLIDOTOMY AND DEEP BRAIN STIMULATION

Treating Parkinson's disease with surgery has once again become more common practice. The basal ganglia nerve cell groups have been the target of both small localised destructive lesions, e.g. in the globus pallidus (pallidotomy), and of deep brain stimulation by electrodes implanted into these areas. Pallidotomy can cause a useful reduction of uncontrollable levodopa-induced dyskinesias and variable improvement in parkinsonism.

Preliminary reports of the effects of deep brain stimulation of the internal globus pallidus and subthalamic nucleus have also been promising. At the six-month follow-up, the severity of the 'off' phase is improved by about one-third, and dyskinesia by about 60 per cent. But, unfortunately, the benefit can wear off after about 6 to 12 months.

The value of chronic bilateral stimulation of the internal globus pallidus and the subthalamic nucleus has been compared in small numbers of patients with young-onset Parkinson's disease. In 'off-drug' phases, the motor score is improved by 70 per cent with subthalamic nucleus stimulation and by 40 per cent with internal globus pallidus stimulation, on average. Although rigidity and tremor show good improvement in both groups, subthalamic nucleus stimulation was better in reducing akinesia. It also allowed a decrease in the levodopa dose of over 50 per cent. The overall results favour the neurosurgical treatment of Parkinson's disease by stimulating the subthalamic nucleus rather than the internal globus pallidus.

NIGRAL TRANSPLANTS

Efforts have been made to replace the damaged dopamine cells by using transplants of other dopaminergic cells in the brain; one source or donor is the dopamine present in a portion of the adrenal glands, sited above the kidneys. More publicity was given to the extension of this work in younger patients in Mexico. This was not a controlled study and the florid publicity in the national press caused more than a little sceptical criticism among neuroscientists worldwide. Isolated reports of similar procedures in North America have confirmed the soundness of this cautious reception. Subsequent operations transplanting the adrenal gland have shown variable and slight benefits. Adrenal gland grafts survive poorly after implantation, but they are capable of inducing sprouting of nerve fibres in the host's caudate nucleus. This approach has been abandoned.

TRANSPLANTATION OF FFETAL TISSUE

Other methods have been attempted, notably the transplantation of substantia nigra from aborted human fetuses. This area is the main focus of loss of dopamine stores in human Parkinson's disease, so it makes good sense to replace it with the same tissue.

CONTINUING PROBLEMS

The number of such operations performed is still small, largely because: it requires major surgery at centres with specialised experience; there are ethical problems in obtaining and using fetal donor tissue; and the long-term benefits are not yet known. The number of patients likely to benefit from current techniques is small.

Strict scientific control comparing cases who have received surgery against those of similar age, sex and severity of illness who have not is essential before we can say that the operation is valuable in certain types or stages of the disease or, conversely, of no benefit to any patient. However, it is encouraging that robust survival of fetal nigral implants can be achieved within the human brain, which can give a new nerve supply to the damaged nerve cells in the basal ganglia.

For the present, these techniques continually advance, but must be viewed with cautious optimism. It is not known whether transplantation alters the progression or outcome of Parkinson's disease. It is not known whether any such benefit will be lasting. It is not known whether those agent(s) that primarily cause the disease will also destroy the graft. We must also remember that Parkinson's disease reflects a disorder not only of dopamine, but of many other neurotransmitters that may not be replaced by the grafts, even if the grafts work. These techniques hold out promise, but we do not know whether they will have a lasting place in the treatment of a small minority of patients. Meanwhile, no patient should feel deprived of an implant until much more research has been completed.

KEY POINTS

✓ Stereotactic surgery can occasionally be beneficial for one-sided shaking and rigidity uncontrollable by drug treatment

✓ Pallidotomy can cause a useful reduction of uncontrollable levodopa-induced dyskinesias and variable improvement in parkinsonism

✓ Preliminary reports of the effects of deep brain stimulation of the internal globus pallidus and subthalamic nucleus have also been promising

✓ Attempts to transplant dopamine-rich fetal tissue into the brains of patients with Parkinson's disease need to be repeated under strictly controlled conditions, before the value of such surgery can be judged

General management

Drug treatment is the most important single measure in reversing the symptoms and disabilities of Parkinson's disease, but there is far more to the treatment of the patient than the administration of drugs alone. Many of the problems faced by patients are not caused by Parkinson's disease itself, but by the coincidental accompanying conditions from which many people suffer and which may need separate medical attention. Some patients are diabetic, some have high blood pressure, some asthma, some heart disease or bronchitis, and many have arthritis. Thus the care of the whole patient is an essential approach from your doctor – GP or specialist.

IDENTIFYING THE PROBLEMS

Certain problems occur commonly in Parkinson's disease and the first step is to identify them. Then, we must outline means of helping to correct them. Here are some common problems in movement you may have noticed, and there are many more:

- walking slowly

- walking with short, shuffling steps

- walking through doorways causing you to stop or hesitate

- freezing of feet to the floor

- turning in a narrow space without falling

- swinging the arms automatically when walking

- getting out of a chair

- standing straight instead of hunched forwards

- turning over in bed

- getting on and off a toilet

- using the hands with fine manipulations, dressing and undressing

- writing smaller, shaky and spidery

- using screwdrivers

- sewing on buttons or crocheting.

PHYSIOTHERAPY

Physiotherapy usually consists of a series of exercise for improving movements and developing function in a compromised part of the body, for example, walking exercises. It has specific benefits for specific problems; it also has a generally beneficial effect in boosting morale, in persuading the patient that something active is being done, and that he or she is playing an active part in the treatment. The motivation, personality and the attitude of both patient and therapist have a marked influence on the general benefits obtained. Bad habits are better eradicated early than late. In advanced illness motivation may be poor, memory and concentration impaired, and effective cooperation may be impossible.

Assessment is the first step. This includes:

- the physical disabilities

- learning capacity and mental state

- home circumstances

- the availability of able-bodied friends and family to continue to practise any instructions.

Exercises

Exercises and activity are important, because they mobilise joints and muscles, lessen stiffness and improve posture. They aim to:

- correct abnormal gait

- correct bad posture

- prevent or minimise stiffness and contractures of the joints

- improve use and facilities of the limbs

- provide a regimen which can be used at home by the patient.

Regular exercise is beneficial whenever disabilities permit. It helps to maintain your muscle tone and strength and helps to prevent contractures and stiffening. Walking is one of the most valuable exercises. Most people in the early stages can walk a mile or two each day, sometimes much more. A conscious effort should be made to keep the back straight, shoulders back, head upright and to take slow, long strides. Even more severe cases can often walk 300 or 400 yards, and perhaps repeat this once or twice every day. Slippery surfaces, snow, ice and wet leaves should obviously be avoided.

The physiotherapist will concentrate on teaching you to sit straight, often in a high upright chair, aided by a cushion in the back.

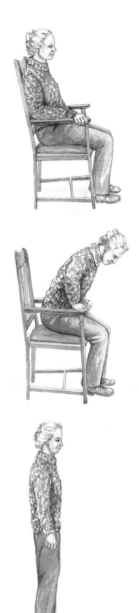

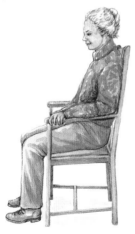

You will be shown how to improve moving from sitting to standing, by pulling your heels in under the front edge of the chair and throwing the weight forward as you get up.

The physiotherapist will show you how to concentrate on striking the heel down when walking,

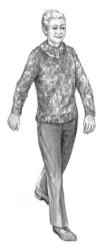

Standing in front of a long mirror may help you to see and correct any stoop or bent posture of the neck and trunk.

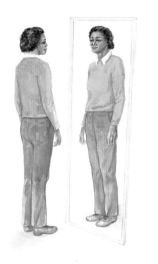

OCCUPATIONAL THERAPY

A wide range of home aids is available, many of which should be available on the NHS, although some may need to be purchased privately. A home visit by an occupational therapist is invaluable, and he or she will usually prepare a report for the hospital consultant describing specific problems, the need for gadgets, hand rails, high seats and other provisions. Wide handles on cutlery, antislip kitchen surfaces, lever arms on taps, raised working surfaces in the kitchen and greenhouse, and Velcro fasteners to garments and shoes are examples of the ways in which you can make your activities and independence easier.

Keep at it

Constant repetition and practice are necessary at home, especially when the therapist is no longer badgering you; there is no substitute for 'do it yourself'! Exercises may be made easier and more rhythmical if performed to music on a cassette, CD or radio. Visits to outpatient therapy may be helpful and encouragement may be obtained by group exercises. Therapeutic holidays, including vigorous activity, can sometimes be arranged (see Useful information on page 60).

Appliances

As the disease progresses, some patients require aids to activity.

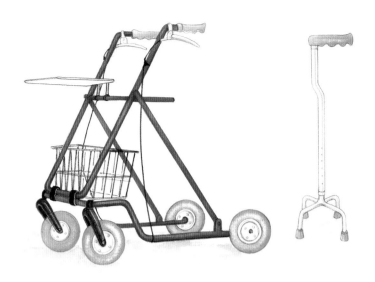

Aids to activity can help to provide a sense of security.

pain of a frozen shoulder – a common complication. Manual dexterity may be improved by practice with blocks, jigsaws and certain games. Grab rails fitted near your bed, in the lavatory and bathroom are helpful. Buttons and zips can be replaced by Velcro fasteners. Casual or elastic sided shoes or trainers may be much easier than lace-up shoes.

Large-handled knives, forks and spoons, stick-on plates and egg cups can save spills. Many of these can be supplied or recommended by the physiotherapist or occupational therapist. The Welfare Department of the Parkinson's Disease Society is also able to advise.

It is of enormous advantage if there is good liaison between the hospital-based physiotherapist, occupational therapist, the social worker and the ward team. They will meet to discuss plans and joint assessments when patients are

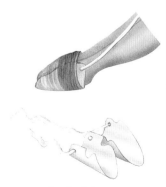

Stocking helper.

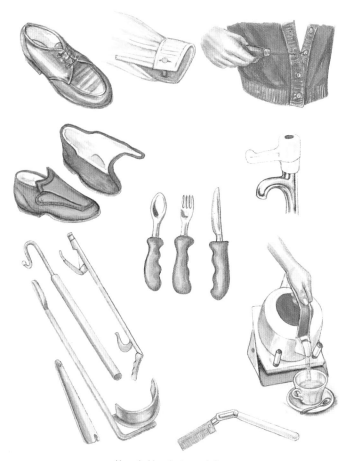

Household gadgets can help.

Walking sticks add to your stability and are socially unobtrusive. A tripod held in one hand does the same thing on a wider base. Zimmer frames are not recommended except as a short-term measure when mobilising after injury or operation in hospital. They break the natural rhythm of walking. If, however, they are fitted with wheels, they are valuable. Delta frames with two 'legs' and a front wheel or a rolator with two legs and two wheels are helpful. Brakes add to your sense of security.

Individual exercises are aimed to help balance, lengthen your stride and perhaps relieve the

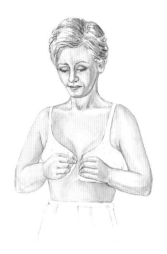

Getting dressed is easier with a bra which fastens at the front.

SPEECH THERAPY

Many patients are embarrassed and frustrated by their speech. You may find that you speak quietly, are unable to shout and that friends are always asking you to repeat yourself, or to speak up, please. Speech may be slurred and hesitant with lack of variation in pitch and volume of the voice. Assessment by a speech therapist will examine the way you breathe, and move your lips, tongue and jaw in the formation of speech – all elements that we do unconsciously or automatically.

In Parkinson's disease, the working of the voice box (larynx) is deficient and produces a monotonous pitch, lack of volume control and lack of stress of certain sounds. Your voice may sound hoarse, quiet and monotonous. Speech therapy

admitted to the ward, and will continue supervision, where possible, after you go home. They will also link up with the GP and district welfare services.

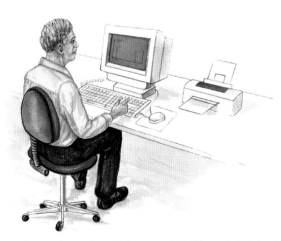

A personal computer can help some patients if finger dexterity is retained.

may use audio feedback in which you hear your own speech after a measured latent interval; this can modify and improve the voice and speech output. This and other manoeuvres can, to a modest extent, help to retrain the voice and speech, but dramatic improvements are not common.

Aids to communication

Communication aids include 'Edu-Com Scanning', a device to point to a word or picture showing your intention and meaning. 'Micro-writer' links a TV, printer or speech synthesiser and can be of occasional help to patients when speech training is unsuccessful. The use of a personal computer (PC) may help you to write letters and perform business activities and attend to your finances from home. Modern programs are fairly easy to learn if you are a newcomer to this tech-nological world; there is a wide range of recreational games and educational material that may occupy and expand your interests.

DIET

Experience has confirmed that eating a well-balanced nutritious diet can be beneficial for anyone. For preventing or curing Parkinson's disease, however, there does not seem to be any specific vitamin, mineral or other nutrient that has any therapeutic value. Sometimes,

a dose of Madopar or Sinemet does not work, particularly with an after-lunch dose. This may occur because proteins in the stomach and intest-ine, from the preceding meal, can interfere with the absorption of the drug into the bloodstream. Your specialist may advise you to have a low-protein lunch with small amounts of meat, fish, poultry, eggs or cheese, but to include these foods in the main evening meal, after which you may not wish to be as active as during the day.

Despite early optimism, it is now well established that vitamin E does not delay Parkinson's disease or its progression.

SOME GENERAL OBSERVATIONS

With the help of your GP you should obtain up-to-date medical support and supervision of your drug and physical treatment, and advice about any possible side effects. More specialised guidance is available from consultants in clinics who should supervise most patients – where staffing levels and facilities permit. The welfare services and hospital units also provide support from physio-therapists, occupational therapists and social workers when the need arises, but currently the provision and quality of support are variable.

Activity throughout the illness is the keynote. Do as much as you can, but be sensible and don't over-do it, to the point of exhaustion. Three walks of 400 yards each are at least as beneficial as one of 1200 yards. You will also have to make certain adjustments to your lifestyle, but these are usually obvious, and changes are gradual so you have plenty of time to make these alterations. You may have to allow a little longer to get dressed or go to work, or to plan and pack for holidays or journeys. It may take two goes to mow the lawn instead of one. Try not to let this irritate you; a little planning, allowing more time, will make most tasks possible.

Don't get fanatical about crack-pot schemes you read about, or about gossip you hear. A lot of money can be wasted on charlatan remedies, health foods, acupunc-ture, osteopathy and so forth. Medical opinion has no rooted objections to these therapies, but does not use them unless they have been carefully and scientifically tested, so that it is clear if they are of benefit or not.

CONCLUSIONS

Although there has been con-siderable progress in the last few years, Parkinson's disease remains something of an enigma. We know that there is degeneration of certain small but vital areas of the brain, but it is not just a condition caused by ageing. Its effects are complex, but the main one is a lack of an essential chemical transmitter, dopamine, which can be effectively replaced by modern drug treat-ment. This permits a full and active life for many years.

The Parkinson's Disease Society and other organisations fund med-ical and social research on a large scale. As a result, there is hardly a year goes by without some important addition to knowledge, additions that are of potential importance to each and every sufferer of the disease.

FUTURE PROSPECTS

To date, there is no way to predict or prevent the disease. However, researchers are looking for a bio-marker – a chemical abnormality that all patients with Parkinson's disease might share – that could be detected by screening techniques or by a simple chemical test given to people who do not have any parkinsonian symptoms.

Positron emission tomography (PET) scanning has yielded advances in our knowledge. PET scans of the brain produce pictures of chem-ical changes as they occur in the living brain. Using PET, scientists can study the brain's dopamine and have shown that it is strik-ingly reduced in the basal ganglia many years before any signs of the disease are apparent. This helps us to understand better the disease process and may lead to improved treatments.

Investigations are proceeding on the role of mitochondria, structures in cells that provide the energy for cellular activity. As MPTP interferes with the function of mitochondria within nerve cells, similar abnormalities may be involved in Parkinson's disease.

Genetic engineering

Scientists are modifying the genetic code of individual cells to attempt to make dopamine-producing cells by using other cells, such as those from the skin. The idea is attractive as a fundamental way of getting at the root cause but, as a practicable treatment, it is still remote.

An array of promising research studies is being done in brain areas other than the substantia nigra, which may be involved in the disease. In laboratory animals, MPTP-induced reduction of dopamine results in overactivity of nerve cells in a region of the brain called the subthalamic nucleus, producing tremors and rigidity, and suggesting that these symptoms may be related to excessive activity in this region. Stimulating or destroying the subthalamic nucleus results in a change of parkinsonian symptoms in the animal models.

'Dopamine transporters' carry dopamine in and out of the narrow gap (synapse) between nerve cells. Investigations have shown a pronounced decline in labelling of striatal dopamine transporters in both early and advanced Parkinson's disease. This decline means that any further threat to the remaining dopamine transporters could contribute to the cause of Parkinson's disease.

Also under investigation are additional controlled-release formulas of Parkinson's disease drugs and implantable pumps that give a continuous supply of levodopa to help patients who have problems with fluctuating levels of response. Another promising treatment method involves implanting capsules containing dopamine-producing cells into the brain.

Tremor control therapy consists of a wire surgically implanted deep within the brain and connected to a pulse generator, similar to a cardiac pacemaker, implanted near the collarbone. Whenever a tremor begins, the patient can activate the device by passing a hand-held magnet over the generator.

The system delivers a mild electrical stimulation that blocks those brain signals that cause tremor. Effects are often dramatic, but much more experience is needed before we know to what extent this system is effective, and for how long.

Questions & answers

● What causes Parkinson's disease?

We don't know the cause. Investigations have sought environmental factors such as contaminants of food, water and air, and exposure to poisonous chemicals at work, but have failed to produce an answer. Although there is a weak hereditary factor, it is not the cause, but may make certain people more susceptible to unidentified substances, to which we may be exposed.

● I have been under a lot of stress. Could that be the cause?

No. Stress and tension may cause a temporary worsening of symptoms, but they do not cause the disease. Depression is a common problem in Parkinson's disease and may reduce your general efficiency, drive and ability to cope. It is generally much improved by antidepressant drugs.

● Will I pass it on to my children or grandchildren?

Although there is a slightly higher incidence of perhaps one in 20 cases in close relatives, Parkinson's disease is not an inherited disease.

● I have heard that Eldepryl (selegiline) will slow down the disease. Should I take it?

Trials in the UK and the USA have now shown that selegiline does not affect the disease process in the brain and has no effect in reducing the rate of progression. It is, nevertheless, useful early in the illness and acts by relieving early symptoms, thereby delaying the time when it is necessary to start levodopa drugs. Side effects are infrequent and usually mild.

● Is there any advantage in delaying the start of levodopa drugs?

As the benefit of levodopa drugs tends to fade after five to ten years, it is generally thought sensible not to start them too soon, that is, before symptoms are of more than nuisance value, and are beginning to interfere with work and leisure. There is no advantage in delaying once this time is reached, and the benefits are usually obvious and will improve your quality of life.

● What will be the effects of levodopa, and will it have side effects?

Within a month or so, stiffness, slowness of movements, walking difficulties and posture start to improve. Shaking does not always disappear, but may be reduced. Benefit continues to increase as the fine tuning of dose and timing is carefully monitored. A few patients have sickness or faintness in the first few weeks, but taking tablets on a full stomach, and starting with small doses that are increased slowly, will allow them

to cope with this. Abnormal movements, fluctuations in effects – before and after each dose – and mental problems can develop later in the illness, but adjustments of drugs and dosage often abolish these symptoms.

● I have taken Madopar (dopamine) for two years. Why am I now getting these funny twitching movements?

These are probably dyskinesias or dystonias caused by a slight overspill or excess of drug on the sensitive receptors in the brain. They usually occur some 30 to 60 minutes after each dose, and last for a few minutes. Your doctor may advise a slight reduction in dose, given at shorter intervals. A controlled-release (CR) preparation helps some patients.

● Why is it taking so long for the tablets to work, and why do they wear off so quickly?

After a few years the body does not absorb or distribute levodopa as efficiently, and the dopamine receptors do not respond quite so effectively, as at the start of treatment. Alteration by your physician of the dose and frequency often improves this problem.

● I find that I can't concentrate or remember things like I used to. Is Parkinson's disease responsible?

Memory and concentration often diminish with normal ageing, irrespective of Parkinson's disease. If you have become depressed, this can also affect concentration and memory, and often improves with simplification of, or additional, drug therapy. A small percentage of Parkinson's disease sufferers become demented.

● Am I likely to benefit from a transplant?

Adrenal transplants are now thought to be ineffective. Fetal transplants are, for the time being, in the experimental stage. They have been shown to be feasible, but their long-term value is not yet established.

Meanwhile, no patient should feel deprived of an implant until we have far more information.

Useful information

ADDRESSES

Parkinson's Disease Society
215 Vauxhall Bridge Road,
London SW1V 1EJ
Helpline: 020 7233 5373 (10am–4pm
Mon–Fri)
Tel: 020 7931 8080
Fax: 020 7233 9908
Website: http://glaxocentre.
merseyside.org/pds.html

Citizens Advice Bureaux
For local information and up-to-date
addresses, see your local telephone
directory.

Disabled Living Foundation
380–384 Harrow Road
London W9 2HU
Helpline: 0870 603 9177
(Minicom 0870 603 9176)
Tel: 020 7289 6111
Email: advice@dlf.org.uk
Website: www.dlf.org.uk

Supports disabled people and their
carers by supplying advice, equipment

and training. Visits by appointment
only for advice about equipment and
appliances.

PUBLICATIONS

There is a useful and regularly updated
selection of books available from the
Parkinson's Disease Society, so contact
them for an up-to-date list – see
address above and useful link to
website below.

USEFUL LINKS

Publications available from the Parkinson's Disease Society
http://glaxocentre.merseyside.org/
booklist2.html

Equipment suppliers
http://www.dlf.org.uk/links/supplier.htm

Disability Net
www.disabilitynet.co.uk
Internet-based disability information
and news services.

Glossary

agonists: agents that drive or stimulate the working of the site or receptor on which they act. By contrast, antagonists block or inhibit function.

akinesia: loss of deliberate voluntary movement.

antagonists: agents that block or inhibit the working of the site or receptor on which they act. See also agonists.

anticholinergic drugs: drugs that oppose acetylcholine, the neurotransmitter which, relative to dopamine, is increased in Parkinson's disease.

arm swing: the ability of the arms to swing naturally and without deliberate attempt during walking.

basal ganglia: large groups of nerve cells deep in the grey matter of the brain.

bilateral: affecting both sides of the body; unilateral means on one side only.

bradykinesia: slowness of movement.

dementia: a decline in intellect, memory and the ability to make rational decisions and judgements.

disorientation: loss of sense of time, place (where you are) and person (who you are).

dopamine: one of a number of transmitters, made in the basal ganglia, and deficient in Parkinson's disease and some related disorders.

dopamine agonists: drugs that drive or stimulate the working of surviving dopamine receptor cells from which dopamine is released.

dopaminergic: dopamine-forming (for example, levodopa) or

dopamine-stimulating, for the receptors (for example, pergolide).

dyskinesia: abnormal movements other than tremor, which in Parkinson's disease is caused by drugs. They are often writhing, twitching or jerking movements.

facies: the appearance of the face often immobile or like a mask in Parkinson's disease.

globus pallidus: one of the pairs of nerve nuclei that make up the basal ganglia.

Lewy bodies: small areas (inclusions) in nerve cells present in practically every Parkinson's disease patient. They appear, under the microscope, as pink blobs, and show a central core with a peripheral halo.

Lewy body disease: a mixture of parkinsonism with dementia in which there is a high density of Lewy bodies, not only in the deep grey matter but also in the mantle or cortex of the brain.

multi-infarct state: this consists of several areas of softening (infarcts) in the brain, the result of multiple strokes. It causes spastic weakness of the limbs and sometimes dementia which may be mistaken for Parkinson's disease.

multi-system atrophy: a disorder in which there are widespread areas of shrinkage of multiple systems of nerve cells in the brain. Parkinsonism is preceded or followed by loss of blood pressure control, sweating and bladder function (autonomic dysfunction).

neurotransmitters: the chemicals (for example, adrenaline, dopamine, acetylcholine) that transmit nerve impulses.

oxidative stress: the release of oxygen compounds (toxic free radicals) by cells which act as a stress that damages cells.

pallidotomy: the surgical destruction of the globus pallidus.

positron emission tomography: a technique using radioactive substances to study the function of the brain.

posture: refers to the position of the body or limbs.

progressive supranuclear palsy: a degenerative condition with limited movements of the eyes, impaired speech and voice as well as parkinsonism.

rigidity: stiffness, a sense of resistance to active movement.

seborrhoea: the greasiness (resulting from secretion from seborrhoeic glands) of the skin seen in some normal people and marked in some patients with Parkinson's disease.

stereotactic surgery: the accurate placement of a lesion by an instrument held in a rigid frame, applied to the skull, fitted with rulers, to locate the target area in three dimensions.

substantia nigra: the black substance forming part of the basal ganglia; it is rich in dopamine cells which connect and drive other parts of the brain to achieve normal movement.

subthalamic nucleus: one of the deeply sited pairs of nerve nuclei that make up the basal ganglia.

transmitters: chemicals that transmit, that is, pass on, a message from one cell to the next, either stimulating or inhibiting the function concerned. It is like electricity which acts as the transmitter of sound waves in the radio.

tremor: shaking, of the limbs or body, at rest, during posture or in movement.

unilateral: affecting one side of the body.

Index